NEW MUM SELF CARE BOOK:

A COMPREHENSIVE GUIDE TO NURTURING A NEW BEGINNING FOR A NEW MUM

CELIA B. DELVALLE

COPYRIGHT

TABLE OF CONTENTS

INTRODUCTION
Welcome to motherhood
Letter to the newborn
About this book

CHAPTER 1:
EMBRACING THE TRANSITION
1.1. Acknowledge the Changes: Understanding the physical, emotional, and lifestyle changes that come with motherhood.
1.2. Setting Realistic Expectations: Embracing the unpredictability and adjusting to the new normal.

CHAPTER 2:
PHYSICAL WELL-BEING
2.1. Postpartum Recovery: Practical advice on recovering from childbirth, healing, and rebuilding strength.
2.2. Nourishing Nutrition: A guide to maintaining a healthy diet to support both your recovery and breastfeeding journey.
2.3. Fitness for New Moms: Gentle exercises to regain strength and boost energy.

CHAPTER 3:
EMOTIONAL WELLNESS

3.1. Managing Postpartum Emotions: Recognizing and coping with the emotional rollercoaster of postpartum life.

3.2. Seeking Support: Building a strong support system, including partner, family, and friends.

3.3. Mental Health: Strategies for maintaining good mental health, including mindfulness and stress management techniques.

CHAPTER 4:
SELF-CARE RITUALS

4.1. Prioritizing "Me Time": Creating space for self-care amidst the demands of motherhood.

4.2. Beauty and Pampering: Simple self-care routines to boost confidence and well-being.

4.3. Sleep Hygiene: Strategies for getting restful sleep and managing sleep deprivation.

CHAPTER 5:
BONDING WITH BABY

5.1. Nurturing Connection: Tips for fostering a strong bond with your newborn.

5.2. Baby Massage and Gentle Activities: Enhancing the bond through soothing touch and engaging activities.

CHAPTER 6:
BALANCING RESPONSIBILITIES

6.1. Time Management: Juggling motherhood, work, and personal time effectively.

6.2. Delegating and Accepting Help: Building a support network and sharing responsibilities.

CHAPTER 7:
RELATIONSHIP DYNAMICS

7.1. Nurturing Your Partnership: Strategies for maintaining a healthy relationship with your partner during this transformative time.

7.2. Communicating Needs: Open communication and understanding each other's roles.

CHAPTER 8:
PLANNING FOR THE FUTURE

8.1. Career and Personal Goals: Balancing motherhood with personal and professional aspirations.

8.2. Long-Term Self-Care: Sustainable practices for ongoing well-being beyond the early postpartum period.

CHAPTER 9:
SLEEP STRATEGIES FOR NEW MOMS

9.1. Tips for optimizing sleep patterns for both you and your baby.

9.2. Coping with sleep deprivation and establishing healthy sleep routines.

9.3. Creating a calming bedtime routine for improved sleep quality.

CHAPTER 10:
ESTABLISHING SELF-CARE ROUTINES

10.1. Developing a personalized self-care plan that fits into your daily life.

10.2. Finding moments for relaxation, mindfulness, and joy amidst the demands of motherhood.

10.3. Balancing the needs of your baby with your own well-being.

INTRODUCTION

WELCOME TO MOTHERHOOD

Congratulations on embarking on the incredible journey of motherhood! Welcome to a chapter of life that is both challenging and profoundly rewarding. As a new mom, you are now part of a community of nurturing, resilient individuals who play a pivotal role in shaping the future.

In these early days, remember to be kind to yourself. Embrace the learning curve, and know that it's okay not to have all the answers. You are navigating uncharted territory, and each day brings new discoveries and joys.

Take the time to savor the precious moments with your little one – the soft coos, the tiny fingers wrapped around yours, and the sweet scent of babyhood. Cherish the quiet moments of bonding as you navigate the intricacies of parenthood.

Lean on your support system; whether it's family, friends, or fellow moms, they can provide valuable insights and a comforting presence. Trust your instincts, for there is no one-size-fits-all manual for motherhood. Your unique connection with your child will guide you through this incredible journey.

As you navigate the challenges and relish the joys, remember that you are not alone. Countless mothers have walked this path before you, and many are walking it alongside you. Embrace the adventure, celebrate the small victories, and know that you are creating a tapestry of love and memories that will last a lifetime. Welcome to the sisterhood of motherhood – a journey filled with boundless love and immeasurable strength.

LETTER TO THE NEWBORN

Hello precious one,

Welcome to the world! Your arrival has filled our hearts with indescribable joy and overwhelming love. From the moment you entered our lives, everything has taken on a new and beautiful meaning.

Tiny fingers, tiny toes, and a heart so pure – you are a miracle, a gift beyond measure. As we hold you close, we promise to cherish and protect you, guiding you through each step of this incredible journey called life.

Your presence has already brought so much light into our lives. Every coo, every smile, and even the late-night cuddles are moments we treasure. We eagerly anticipate watching you grow, learn, and discover the wonders of the world.

Know that you are surrounded by love, warmth, and endless support. We are here to nurture, encourage, and be your steadfast companions. Your journey is our journey, and we are grateful to share it with you.

May your days be filled with laughter, your dreams be boundless, and your heart always know the profound love that surrounds you. Welcome to our family, sweet one. You are our greatest blessing.

With all our love,
Your Mum

ABOUT THIS BOOK

This book, **"NEW MUM SELF CARE BOOK**: A comprehensive guide to nurturing a new beginning for a new mum." is a heartfelt companion crafted for the incredible women stepping into the transformative realm of motherhood. As you embark on this beautiful journey, we recognize the myriad emotions, challenges, and joys that come with the arrival of a new life.

In these pages, you'll find more than just practical advice; you'll discover a holistic approach to self-care that goes beyond the surface, delving into the physical, emotional, and relational facets of your new role. "NEW MUM SELF CARE BOOK" is designed to empower you to prioritize your well-being, fostering not only a resilient and confident new mother but also a nurturing environment for your precious little one.

This guide is a roadmap through the ups and downs, offering insights into postpartum recovery, emotional wellness, self-care rituals, and the delicate art of balancing responsibilities. Whether you're a first-time mum or adding another member to your growing family, these pages are filled with wisdom, support, and practical strategies to help you navigate this unique and transformative time.

So, dear reader, let the journey begin. May this book be a source of comfort, inspiration, and empowerment as you embark on the beautiful adventure of motherhood. Here's to nurturing new beginnings and celebrating the incredible woman you are becoming.

CHAPTER 1:
EMBRACING THE TRANSITION

1.1. ACKNOWLEDGING THE CHANGES

The journey into motherhood is a profound transition that unfolds with a tapestry of changes – physical, emotional, and lifestyle. As you cradle your newborn in your arms, it's essential to acknowledge and understand the shifts that have occurred within you and around you.

- **A Symphony Of Physical Changes:**

The journey into motherhood orchestrates a profound symphony of physical changes, each note resonating with the extraordinary process of bringing life into the world. Your body, a marvel of nature, undergoes a transformative performance, reflecting the strength, adaptability, and resilience inherent in the female form.

- **Miracle of Childbirth:**

The overture to this symphony is the miracle of childbirth. The crescendo of labor, the rhythm of contractions, and the breathtaking moment of delivery compose a melody that echoes the power within you. Embrace the physical intensity of childbirth as a testament to your body's innate ability to nurture and bring forth life.

- **Postpartum Recovery:**

As the curtains fall on the delivery stage, the postpartum period takes center stage. This movement involves the delicate process of recovery—physically and emotionally. Acknowledge the changes, whether it's the tender healing of stitches or the recalibration of hormonal balances. This is a period of regeneration, a time for your body to convalesce and renew.

- **Nourishing and Adapting:**

The intermezzo of breastfeeding and nourishing your newborn introduces a harmonious element to the symphony. Your body adapts to provide sustenance, embracing the profound connection forged during those quiet moments of feeding.

Recognize the beauty in this symbiotic relationship, understanding that your body is a source of comfort, nourishment, and warmth for your little one.

- **Physical Resilience:**

Every stretch mark, scar, or change in physique is a note in the symphony of physical resilience. Your body, marked by the journey of motherhood, becomes a living testament to the challenges overcome and the beauty created. Celebrate these physical manifestations as a reflection of the strength and endurance that define the maternal experience.

- **Culmination of Transformation:**

As the symphony reaches its finale, the culmination of physical changes paints a portrait of transformation. Your body, once solely yours, now carries the imprints of the extraordinary feat of childbirth. Embrace this metamorphosis with a sense of awe and gratitude, recognizing that every change signifies the emergence of a new chapter in your life.

In acknowledging the symphony of physical changes, you honor the unique composition that is your journey into motherhood. Each movement, whether powerful or delicate, contributes to the masterpiece that is your story. Embrace the physical changes as a symphony of strength, resilience, and the enduring beauty of the maternal experience.

- **The Landscape Of Emotions:**

Motherhood is a profound journey that traverses a vast and intricate landscape of emotions. The emotional spectrum, much like the changing seasons, encompasses a myriad of feelings that ebb and flow, creating a tapestry unique to each individual. In navigating this emotional terrain, acknowledging and embracing the diversity of your feelings is key to understanding the depth and richness of the maternal experience.

- **Overwhelming Love:**

At the heart of this emotional landscape is the overwhelming love that engulfs you upon meeting your newborn. It is a love so profound, so all-encompassing, that it reshapes your very being. Embrace this love without reservation, recognizing it as the foundation upon which the bond with your child will flourish.

- **Joy and Happiness:**

Among the hills and valleys of motherhood, you will encounter moments of unbridled joy and happiness. From the first smile of your baby to the shared laughter that fills your home, relish these moments as the purest expressions of happiness. Allow them to uplift your spirit and illuminate the path ahead.

- **Occasional Doubt:**

In the shadows of joy, occasional doubt may cast its fleeting presence. It is natural to question your abilities and decisions. Acknowledge these doubts with compassion, understanding that they are part of the intricate dance of learning and growing as a mother. Seek support and trust in your resilience.

- **Moments of Exhaustion:**

The emotional landscape also features moments of exhaustion, where the demands of motherhood may seem overwhelming. It's crucial to recognize and address these feelings, ensuring that self-care becomes a priority. Embrace the importance of rest, seeking solace in moments of quiet reflection.

- **Vulnerability and Sensitivity:**

Motherhood often unveils a heightened sense of vulnerability and sensitivity. The world may feel more poignant, emotions more acute. Embrace this sensitivity as a source of strength, allowing yourself to connect deeply with your child and your own inner self.

- **Navigating the Unexpected:**

The landscape of emotions is not always predictable. Unexpected challenges may arise, stirring emotions you hadn't anticipated. Embrace the uncertainty, understanding that navigating the unexpected is a testament to your adaptability and resilience.

In acknowledging the diverse emotions that color your maternal journey, you cultivate emotional intelligence and resilience. Each feeling, whether light or heavy, joyous or challenging, is a brushstroke on the canvas of your motherhood. Embrace this emotional landscape as an integral part of the transformative journey you are undertaking—one that adds depth, meaning, and unparalleled richness to your role as a mother.

1.2. SETTING REALISTIC EXPECTATIONS

Amidst the awe-inspiring journey of motherhood, setting realistic expectations becomes a guiding compass, steering you through the unpredictable seas of change. This chapter is a gentle reminder that the path you walk is uniquely yours, and by embracing flexibility and authenticity, you pave the way for a more fulfilling and compassionate motherhood experience.

- **The Unpredictable Nature of New Motherhood:**

Motherhood is an adventure, and adventures are known for their unpredictability. The first step in setting realistic expectations is acknowledging that each baby is unique, and there's no one-size-fits-all manual. Embrace spontaneity and understand that flexibility is your greatest ally. Your baby's needs and rhythms may not conform to a predetermined schedule, and that's perfectly normal.

- **Adapting to the New Normal:**

As you transition into motherhood, it's essential to redefine what "normal" means for you. Your routine and lifestyle will undergo changes, and embracing these adjustments can make the journey smoother. Setting realistic expectations involves understanding that your daily life may look different now, and that's not only okay but a natural part of the transformative process.

- **Honoring Individual Experiences:**
Comparisons can be a thief of joy. Setting realistic expectations requires embracing the uniqueness of your journey. Resist the temptation to measure your experience against others. Every mother and every baby is on a distinct path. Your challenges, triumphs, and pace of adaptation are individual, and by honoring these differences, you free yourself from unnecessary pressure.

- **Embracing the Spontaneity:**
While routines can be beneficial, setting realistic expectations involves embracing the beauty in spontaneity. Be open to the unexpected and find joy in the unplanned moments. This mindset shift allows you to appreciate the nuances of motherhood without feeling burdened by rigid expectations.

- **Flexibility as a Strength:**
In the world of motherhood, flexibility is not a sign of weakness but a display of strength. Setting realistic expectations means

understanding that plans may change, and that's okay. Give yourself permission to adapt, pivot, and find joy in the fluidity of the journey.

- **Cultivating Patience:**

Setting realistic expectations requires a dose of patience. Whether it's in understanding your baby's cues or adapting to your evolving identity, patience becomes a valuable ally. Recognize that the journey unfolds gradually, and every challenge is an opportunity for growth.

In setting realistic expectations, you create a foundation for a more balanced and enjoyable motherhood experience. Embrace the unpredictability, redefine your normal, and celebrate the unique journey you are on. By doing so, you cultivate a mindset that not only enhances your well-being but also allows you to savor the beauty in every moment of this transformative adventure.

In this chapter, we lay the foundation for a mindful and compassionate approach to the transition into motherhood. By acknowledging the changes and setting realistic expectations, you pave the way for a journey that is uniquely yours – one filled with discovery, growth, and the profound joy of nurturing new beginnings.

CHAPTER 2:
PHYSICAL WELL-BEING

2.1. POSTPARTUM RECOVERY:

Practical advice on recovering from childbirth, healing, and rebuilding strength.

The postpartum period, often referred to as the "fourth trimester," is a critical time of adjustment and recovery for both the mother and the newborn. This phase, typically spanning the first six weeks after childbirth, involves physical, emotional, and lifestyle changes.

The postpartum period is a time of physical recovery, emotional adjustment, and establishing new routines. It's a phase that requires understanding, support, and self-care to navigate the challenges and celebrate the joys that come with the arrival of a new family member. Seeking guidance from healthcare professionals and building a support system are integral components of a positive postpartum experience.

This period is a delicate and transformative phase that requires careful attention to your physical and emotional well-being. This chapter offers practical advice on postpartum recovery, guiding you through the journey of healing and rebuilding strength as you embrace the beautiful challenges of early motherhood.

- **Prioritizing Rest and Sleep:**

In the midst of caring for your newborn, prioritizing rest and sleep is paramount. Adequate sleep not only accelerates physical healing but also supports emotional well-being. Create a sleep-friendly environment, nap when your baby naps, and lean on your support system to ensure you get the rest your body craves.

- **Nutrient-Rich Diet:**

Fueling your body with a nutrient-rich diet is crucial for postpartum recovery. Focus on foods that support healing, such as lean proteins, fruits, vegetables, and whole grains. Hydration is equally important, especially if you're breastfeeding. Consult with your healthcare provider about any necessary supplements to complement your diet.

- **Gentle Exercise and Movement:**
Engage in gentle exercises to aid in the recovery process. Start with pelvic floor exercises and gradually incorporate low-impact activities like walking and postpartum yoga. Listen to your body, and avoid high-impact workouts until you've received the green light from your healthcare provider. Exercise can enhance both physical and emotional well-being.

- **Pelvic Floor Care:**
Pay special attention to your pelvic floor, which undergoes significant stress during childbirth. Pelvic floor exercises, known as Kegels, can help strengthen these muscles. Additionally, consider consulting with a pelvic health physical therapist for personalized guidance on pelvic floor care and recovery.

- **Seeking Professional Guidance:**

Regular check-ups with your healthcare provider are crucial for monitoring your postpartum recovery. Share any concerns or discomfort you may be experiencing, and work collaboratively to address them. Your healthcare provider can offer guidance on issues such as pain management, incision care (if applicable), and overall recovery progress.

- **Embracing Emotional Well-Being:**

Postpartum recovery extends beyond the physical realm; it involves nurturing your emotional well-being. Communicate openly with your partner, family, and friends about your emotions. If you're experiencing symptoms of postpartum mood disorders, such as anxiety or depression, seek professional support promptly. Mental well-being is an integral part of the recovery process.

- **Connect with Other Moms:**

Building a community of fellow moms can be invaluable during postpartum recovery. Share experiences, tips, and support with those who understand the unique challenges of early motherhood. Joining postpartum support groups or online communities can provide a sense of camaraderie and encouragement.

Gradual Return to Activities:

As your body heals, gradually reintroduce activities that bring you joy. Whether it's gentle exercises, hobbies, or socializing, listen to your body's cues and pace yourself. Balancing self-care with the demands of motherhood is an ongoing process, and it's essential to be patient with yourself as you navigate this journey.

In prioritizing postpartum recovery, you honor the resilience of your body and spirit. This chapter encourages a holistic approach to healing, recognizing that both physical and emotional well-being are integral to the transformative experience of early motherhood.

2.2. NOURISHING NUTRITION:

A guide to maintaining a healthy diet to support both your recovery and breastfeeding journey.

As a new mother, nourishing your body with a wholesome and balanced diet is not only essential for your postpartum recovery but also plays a pivotal role in supporting a healthy breastfeeding journey. This chapter provides a comprehensive guide to maintaining a nutritious diet that fosters your well-being and provides optimal nutrition for both you and your baby.

- **Hydration: The Foundation of Well-Being**

Start with the simplest yet most crucial element—hydration. Adequate water intake is vital, especially during breastfeeding. Aim to drink at least 8 cups of water per day, and increase this amount if you're physically active or in a warmer climate. Herbal teas and water-rich foods like fruits and vegetables can also contribute to your overall hydration.

- **Balanced Nutrition for Recovery:**

Your body requires a variety of nutrients for effective recovery post childbirth. Focus on a balanced diet that includes:

1. **PROTEINS**:

Essential for tissue repair and muscle recovery. Sources include lean meats, poultry, fish, eggs, dairy, legumes, and plant-based proteins like tofu and tempeh.

Protein is a crucial nutrient for new moms as it supports postpartum recovery, helps with tissue repair, and provides the energy needed for the demands of motherhood. Here are some protein-rich food sources that can benefit new mothers:

- **<u>Lean Meats</u>**: Incorporate lean meats such as chicken, turkey, and lean cuts of beef. These are excellent sources of high-quality protein.

- **Fish:** Opt for fatty fish like salmon, which not only provides protein but also delivers omega-3 fatty acids that support brain and eye health.

- **Eggs**: Eggs are a versatile and nutritious protein source. They contain essential amino acids and various vitamins and minerals.

- **Dairy Products**: Include dairy products like yogurt, milk, and cheese for a good dose of protein and calcium, which is essential for bone health.

- **Legumes**: Beans, lentils, and chickpeas are rich in protein, fiber, and various vitamins and minerals. They are versatile and can be included in a variety of dishes.

- **Tofu and Tempeh:** These plant-based protein sources are excellent alternatives for those following a vegetarian or vegan diet. They can be used in a variety of dishes and provide a good amount of protein.

- **<u>Nuts and Seeds:</u>** Almonds, peanuts, chia seeds, and flaxseeds are protein-packed and provide healthy fats. They make for convenient and nutritious snacks.

- **<u>Quinoa</u>**: Quinoa is a grain that is also a complete protein, meaning it contains all essential amino acids. It can be a great addition to salads, bowls, or as a side dish.

- **<u>Greek Yogurt</u>**: Greek yogurt is a dairy product that is higher in protein compared to regular yogurt. It also contains probiotics, which can be beneficial for gut health.

- **<u>Protein Supplements:</u>** In some cases, new moms may find it challenging to meet their protein needs through food alone. In such instances, protein supplements like whey protein powder can be considered, but it's crucial to consult with a healthcare provider before adding supplements.

Remember to maintain a balanced diet and choose a variety of protein sources to ensure you're getting a broad spectrum of nutrients. If you have specific dietary considerations or restrictions, consult with a healthcare professional or a registered dietitian to create a personalized nutrition plan that meets your individual needs.

2. FRUITS AND VEGETABLES:

Packed with vitamins, minerals, and antioxidants crucial for healing. Aim for a colorful variety to ensure a diverse range of nutrients.

Including a variety of fruits and vegetables in the diet of a new mom is essential for providing a range of vitamins, minerals, and antioxidants that support overall health and postpartum recovery. Here are some fruits and vegetables beneficial for new mothers:

FRUITS:

- **<u>Berries (Blueberries, Strawberries, Raspberries):</u>** Rich in antioxidants and vitamins, berries provide a burst of flavor and can be added to yogurt, smoothies, or enjoyed as a snack.

- **<u>Bananas:</u>** High in potassium and easy to incorporate into various dishes or eaten on their own, bananas are a convenient and energy-boosting fruit.

- **<u>Citrus Fruits (Oranges, Grapefruits, Clementines):</u>** Packed with vitamin C, citrus fruits aid in immune function and collagen production. They can be enjoyed fresh or as part of a fruit salad.

- **<u>Avocado:</u>** A nutrient-dense fruit, avocados provide healthy fats, fiber, and various vitamins. They are a versatile addition to salads, sandwiches, or as a spread.

- **Kiwi:** Kiwi is a good source of vitamin C, vitamin K, and dietary fiber. It adds a refreshing touch to fruit salads or can be eaten on its own.

- **Apples:** High in fiber and a variety of nutrients, apples make for a convenient and satisfying snack. Pair them with nut butter for added protein.

VEGETABLES:
- **Leafy Greens (Spinach, Kale, Swiss Chard):**Packed with iron, calcium, and vitamins, leafy greens support energy levels and overall well-being. They can be added to salads, smoothies, or sautéed as a side dish.

- **Broccoli:** A rich source of vitamins C and K, as well as fiber, broccoli can be steamed, roasted, or added to stir-fries for a nutritious boost.

- **<u>Sweet Potatoes:</u>** High in beta-carotene and fiber, sweet potatoes provide a delicious and nutrient-dense option. Roast, mash, or use them in soups.

- **<u>Bell Peppers:</u>** Rich in vitamin C and antioxidants, bell peppers can be added to salads, stir-fries, or enjoyed as a crunchy snack with hummus.

- **<u>Carrots:</u>** Carrots are a good source of beta-carotene, which is important for eye health. They can be enjoyed raw, roasted, or added to soups and stews.

- **<u>Tomatoes:</u>** Tomatoes are rich in antioxidants like lycopene. They can be used fresh in salads, cooked in sauces, or enjoyed as a snack.

Remember to aim for a colorful variety of fruits and vegetables to ensure a broad spectrum of nutrients. Including these in your diet will not only support your postpartum recovery but also contribute to your overall health and well-being.

3. **WHOLE GRAINS**:

Provide energy and are a good source of fiber. Opt for whole grains like brown rice, quinoa, oats, and whole wheat.

Including whole grains in the diet of a new mom is a great way to provide essential nutrients, fiber, and sustained energy. Here are some wholesome grains that can be beneficial:

- **<u>Quinoa</u>**: A complete protein source, quinoa is versatile and can be used in salads, bowls, or as a side dish. It's rich in fiber, vitamins, and minerals.

- **<u>Brown Rice:</u>** A good source of complex carbohydrates, brown rice provides energy and is high in fiber. It can be used as a base for various dishes.

- **<u>Oats</u>**: Oats are rich in soluble fiber, promoting digestive health. They can be enjoyed as oatmeal, added to smoothies, or used in baking.

- **<u>Barley</u>**: Barley is a hearty grain high in fiber and certain vitamins. It can be used in soups, stews, or as a side dish.

- **<u>Whole Wheat:</u>** Choose whole wheat bread, pasta, and tortillas for added fiber. They can be included in sandwiches, wraps, or pasta dishes.

- **<u>Quinoa Pasta:</u>** A gluten-free alternative to traditional pasta, quinoa pasta provides a good source of protein and can be used in various pasta dishes.

- **<u>Buckwheat</u>**: Despite its name, buckwheat is gluten-free and rich in protein. It can be used in porridge, pancakes, or as a base for salads.

- **<u>Farro</u>**: Farro is an ancient grain that is high in fiber and protein. It has a nutty flavor and can be used in salads, soups, or as a side dish.

- **<u>Millet:</u>** Millet is a gluten-free grain rich in magnesium and phosphorus. It can be used in pilafs, porridge, or as a side dish.

- **<u>Whole Wheat Couscous:</u>** Couscous made from whole wheat provides more fiber than traditional couscous. It's quick to prepare and can be used as a base for various dishes.

Including a variety of these whole grains in your diet not only supports your nutritional needs but also helps in maintaining steady energy levels, promoting digestive health, and providing essential vitamins and minerals. Be sure to balance these grains with a variety of other nutrient-rich foods for a well-rounded and nourishing postpartum diet.

4. HEALTHY FATS:

Support hormonal balance and brain function. Incorporate sources such as avocados, nuts, seeds, and olive oil.

Incorporating healthy fats into the diet of a new mom is crucial for various aspects of postpartum health, including energy, hormone production, and overall well-being. Here are some sources of healthy fats to consider:

- **<u>Avocado</u>**: Packed with monounsaturated fats, avocados also provide fiber and various vitamins. Enjoy them sliced on toast, in salads, or blended into smoothies.

- **<u>Olive Oil:</u>** Extra virgin olive oil is a source of monounsaturated fats and antioxidants. Use it in salad dressings, for sautéing, or drizzle it over cooked dishes.

- **<u>Fatty Fish (Salmon, Mackerel, Trout):</u>** Rich in omega-3 fatty acids, fatty fish support brain health and can positively impact mood. Aim for at least two servings of fatty fish per week.

- **Nuts and Seeds (Almonds, Walnuts, Chia Seeds):** These are excellent sources of healthy fats, as well as protein and essential nutrients. Include them in snacks, sprinkle on yogurt, or add to smoothies.

- **Coconut Oil:** While high in saturated fats, coconut oil contains medium-chain triglycerides (MCTs) that may have health benefits. Use it in moderation for cooking or as an ingredient in certain dishes.

- **Flaxseeds**: Rich in alpha-linolenic acid (ALA), a type of omega-3 fatty acid, flaxseeds can be added to oatmeal, yogurt, or smoothies for a nutritional boost.

- **Chia Seeds**: These tiny seeds are rich in omega-3 fatty acids, fiber, and antioxidants. Mix them into yogurt, make chia pudding, or add to beverages.

- **<u>Dark Chocolate</u>**: Choose dark chocolate with a high cocoa content for a source of monounsaturated fats and antioxidants. Enjoy it in moderation as a satisfying treat.

- **<u>Nut Butters (Peanut Butter, Almond Butter):</u>** These spreads are rich in healthy fats and can be added to toast, used in smoothies, or enjoyed with fruit.

- **<u>Seaweed and Algae:</u>** Certain seaweeds and algae supplements provide omega-3 fatty acids, especially DHA, which is important for brain health. Consult with a healthcare professional before adding supplements.

Remember that while healthy fats are beneficial, moderation is key. Balancing these fats with a variety of nutrient-dense foods will contribute to a well-rounded and nourishing postpartum diet. Always consult with your healthcare provider or a registered dietitian for personalized dietary advice based on your specific needs and health status.

5. DAIRY OR CALCIUM ALTERNATIVES:

Essential for bone health. Include dairy products, fortified plant-based milk, or other calcium-rich foods.

Ensuring an adequate intake of calcium is important for new moms, especially for bone health and overall well-being. If you're lactose intolerant, have dietary restrictions, or choose not to consume dairy, there are alternative sources of calcium to consider:

- **<u>Fortified Plant-Based Milk (Almond, Soy, Coconut, Oat):</u>** Many plant-based milk alternatives are fortified with calcium and vitamin D. Choose unsweetened varieties for a lower sugar content.

- **<u>Fortified Orange Juice:</u>** Some brands of orange juice are fortified with calcium and vitamin D. Check the labels to ensure you are choosing a fortified option.

- **<u>Leafy Green Vegetables (Kale, Broccoli, Bok Choy):</u>** These vegetables are good sources of calcium. Include a variety of leafy greens in your meals, either raw in salads or cooked in stir-fries and soups.

- **<u>Tofu and Tempeh</u>**: These plant-based protein sources also contain calcium. Use them in stir-fries, salads, or marinate and grill for added flavor.

- **<u>Canned Fish with Bones (Salmon, Sardines):</u>** Certain fish, especially those canned with bones, provide not only calcium but also omega-3 fatty acids.

Include them in salads or enjoy whole-grain crackers.

- **<u>Chia Seeds:</u>** In addition to being a good source of healthy fats, chia seeds contain calcium. Mix them into yogurt, smoothies, or make chia pudding.

- **<u>Almonds and Almond Butter:</u>** Almonds are a source of calcium and can be enjoyed as a snack or added to various dishes. Almond butter is another option to spread on whole-grain toast or use in recipes.

- **<u>Fortified Breakfast Cereals:</u>** Some breakfast cereals are fortified with calcium and other nutrients. Choose whole-grain, low-sugar options for a nutritious start to your day.

- **<u>Fortified Non-Dairy Yogurts:</u>** If you prefer non-dairy alternatives, look for yogurts made from almond, coconut, or soy that are fortified with calcium.

- **<u>Calcium Supplements:</u>** In consultation with your healthcare provider, you may consider calcium supplements to ensure you meet your daily requirements. It's essential to get professional advice to determine the right dosage for your specific needs.

Remember to focus on a balanced and varied diet that includes a mix of these calcium-rich alternatives. If you have specific dietary concerns or health conditions, consult with a healthcare professional or a registered dietitian to ensure you are meeting your nutritional needs during the postpartum period.

- **Breastfeeding-specific Nutrients:**

If you're breastfeeding, certain nutrients become even more critical:

-**Calcium**: Necessary for your baby's bone development. Include dairy, fortified plant-based milk, and leafy greens.

-**Iron**: Vital for both you and your baby's blood health. Lean meats, beans, lentils, and fortified cereals are excellent sources.

-**Omega-3 Fatty Acids:** Found in fatty fish, flaxseeds, chia seeds, and walnuts. These support your baby's brain development.

-**Folate**: Important for cell division and DNA synthesis. Leafy greens, citrus fruits, and fortified grains are good sources.

- **Meal Planning for Convenience:**
Given the demands of motherhood, prioritize convenience without compromising nutrition. Prepare simple, nutritious meals in advance, and consider healthy snacks for quick energy boosts. This approach ensures you have easy access to nourishing food, supporting your overall well-being.

- **Supplementation Guidance:**

While a balanced diet is the primary goal, your healthcare provider may recommend supplements to fill potential nutritional gaps. Common supplements for new mothers include prenatal vitamins, vitamin D, and omega-3 fatty acids.

- **Listening to Your Body:**

Finally, tune in to your body's cues. Eat when you're hungry, and pay attention to cravings. Incorporate a variety of foods, and don't be too restrictive. Nourishing your body is a dynamic process, and flexibility is key.

By adopting a mindful and balanced approach to nutrition, you empower your body to recover effectively and provide optimal nourishment for your breastfeeding journey. This chapter encourages you to view food as a source of healing and strength, embracing the transformative power of a well-nourished body during this significant chapter of motherhood.

3.3. FITNESS FOR NEW MOMS:

Gentle exercises to regain strength and boost energy.

Embarking on a fitness routine as a new mom is a gentle yet impactful way to regain strength, boost energy levels, and support overall well-being. This chapter introduces a range of gentle exercises tailored for the postpartum period, ensuring a gradual and enjoyable return to physical activity.

- **Pelvic Floor Exercises (Kegels):**

Start with pelvic floor exercises to rebuild strength in the pelvic region. Kegels involve contracting and relaxing the pelvic floor muscles. Perform these exercises regularly to enhance pelvic stability and support bladder control.

- **Postpartum Yoga:**

Explore postpartum yoga, a gentle practice that combines breath with movement. Yoga helps improve flexibility, core strength, and overall body awareness. Seek out classes specifically designed for postpartum recovery or follow online videos that cater to new moms.

- **Walking**:

A simple yet effective exercise, walking is ideal for gradually reintroducing physical activity. Begin with short walks around your neighborhood, gradually increasing the duration as you feel more comfortable. This low-impact exercise not only boosts energy but also provides a refreshing change of scenery.

- **Bodyweight Exercises:**

Incorporate bodyweight exercises that target major muscle groups. Squats, lunges, and modified push-ups are excellent choices. These exercises help strengthen your legs, glutes, and upper body, promoting overall muscle tone.

- **Low-Impact Cardio:**

Engage in low-impact cardio exercises such as swimming or stationary cycling. These activities provide a cardiovascular workout without putting excessive strain on joints. Adjust the intensity based on your comfort level and gradually increase as your fitness improves.

- **Core Strengthening:**

Focus on rebuilding core strength with exercises like pelvic tilts, gentle abdominal contractions, and modified planks. These exercises contribute to postpartum abdominal recovery, especially if you've experienced diastasis recti.

- **Mom and Baby Workouts:**

Incorporate your little one into your fitness routine with mom and baby workouts. These may include baby-wearing exercises, stroller walks, or gentle movements that involve your baby. Not only does this allow for bonding time, but it also adds an element of fun to your workouts.

- **Flexibility Training:**

Prioritize flexibility with stretching exercises. Incorporate dynamic stretches to improve range of motion and static stretches to enhance flexibility. Stretching can alleviate muscle tension and contribute to a sense of relaxation.

- **Listen to Your Body:**

Above all, listen to your body throughout your fitness journey. Pay attention to how you feel during and after exercises. If an activity causes discomfort or pain, modify or skip it. Gradual progression is key, and patience is your ally in rebuilding strength postpartum.

- **Consult with a Professional:**

Before starting any fitness routine, consult with your healthcare provider. They can provide personalized guidance based on your individual recovery and ensure that your chosen exercises are safe and suitable for your postpartum journey.

Embracing fitness as a new mom is a holistic approach to self-care. These gentle exercises are designed to empower you, promoting physical well-being while respecting the unique demands of the postpartum period. Enjoy the process, celebrate your progress, and savor the rejuvenating benefits of incorporating movement into your new mom routine.

As we draw the curtain on this chapter devoted to physical well-being, we've explored the multifaceted journey of postpartum recovery, nourishing nutrition, and gentle fitness for new moms. These pillars collectively form a foundation for holistic self-care, supporting your body and spirit during this transformative period.

Postpartum Recovery has been a guide through the intricate process of healing after childbirth. From prioritizing rest and hydration to incorporating gentle exercises and seeking professional guidance, it underscores the importance of giving your body the time and care it needs to recover fully.

Nourishing Nutrition has provided a roadmap for maintaining a healthy diet tailored to support both your recovery and breastfeeding journey. Embracing a balance of proteins, fruits, vegetables, whole grains, and essential nutrients is not just about fueling your body but also nurturing your baby through breastfeeding.

Fitness for New Moms has introduced a gentle and gradual approach to physical activity. From pelvic floor exercises to postpartum yoga and mom-and-baby workouts, these exercises are designed to rebuild strength and boost energy without overwhelming your postpartum body.

In the intersection of these three elements, we find a harmonious symphony of self-care. Postpartum recovery, nourishing nutrition, and fitness create a holistic framework that acknowledges the unique needs of new mothers. It's a journey of rediscovery, where your body, after the incredible feat of childbirth, is supported and nurtured to regain strength and vitality.

As you navigate this chapter, remember that there is no one-size-fits-all approach. Each woman's postpartum experience is as unique as her fingerprint. Be patient with yourself, celebrate small victories, and lean into the support of healthcare professionals, loved ones, and the wider community of new moms.

In embracing the practical advice, nutritional guidance, and gentle exercises offered in this chapter, you are not just nurturing physical well-being but weaving a tapestry of resilience, self-love, and empowerment. Here's to your continued journey of thriving physical health and well-being as you embrace the beautiful challenges and joys of new motherhood.

CHAPTER 3:
EMOTIONAL WELLNESS

Welcome to the exploration of emotional wellness, a chapter dedicated to nurturing the intricate landscape of your emotions during the transformative journey of motherhood. This section delves into strategies and insights that empower you to navigate the emotional nuances with resilience, self-compassion, and a deep understanding of the emotional tapestry that unfolds during this special chapter of life.

3.1. MANAGING POSTPARTUM EMOTIONS:

Recognizing and coping with the emotional rollercoaster of postpartum life.

The postpartum period is a time of profound emotional shifts, and managing these emotions is integral to your overall well-being. This section provides practical guidance on navigating the complexities of postpartum emotions, fostering resilience, and embracing a positive emotional landscape.

- **Acknowledging a Spectrum of Emotions:**

Recognize that the postpartum journey encompasses a spectrum of emotions. From joy and love to occasional doubt or anxiety, each feeling is valid and part of the natural tapestry of motherhood. Allow yourself the space to experience and express these emotions without judgment.

- **Cultivating Self-Compassion:**

Practice self-compassion as you navigate the challenges of new motherhood. Understand that it's okay not to have all the answers and that imperfections are a part of the journey. Treat yourself with the same kindness and understanding you would offer a dear friend.

- **Building a Support System:**

Surround yourself with a supportive network of family, friends, and fellow moms. Share your emotions openly, and lean on your support system when needed. Knowing you're not alone in your experiences can be immensely comforting and validating.

- **Prioritizing Self-Care:**

Prioritize self-care as a non-negotiable aspect of managing postpartum emotions. Establish self-care rituals that nurture your emotional well-being, whether it's taking short breaks, indulging in hobbies, or simply enjoying moments of quiet reflection. Remember that caring for yourself enhances your ability to care for your baby.

- **Mindfulness and Relaxation Techniques:**

Incorporate mindfulness and relaxation techniques into your daily routine. Practices such as deep breathing, meditation, or gentle yoga can help center your mind, alleviate stress, and create a sense of calm amid the demands of motherhood.

- **Effective Time Management:**

Managing postpartum emotions is closely tied to effective time management. Prioritize tasks, delegate when possible, and set realistic expectations for yourself. Balancing responsibilities allows for a smoother emotional journey as you navigate the challenges of daily life with a newborn.

- **Communication with Your Partner:**

Open communication with your partner is crucial. Share your emotions, fears, and joys openly. Your partner can be a valuable source of support and understanding, strengthening your connection during this transformative time.

- **Seeking Professional Support:**

If your emotions become overwhelming or if you're experiencing symptoms of postpartum mood disorders, don't hesitate to seek professional support. Mental health professionals specializing in maternal well-being can provide guidance, counseling, and support tailored to your unique situation.

- **Journaling and Reflection:**

Consider keeping a journal to express your thoughts and emotions. Journaling provides a reflective outlet, allowing you to process your experiences and gain insights into your emotional landscape. It can be a therapeutic practice that enhances self-awareness.

- **Connecting with Other Moms:**

Joining mom groups, whether in-person or online, provides a space for shared experiences. Connecting with other moms fosters a sense of community, and knowing that others are facing similar emotions can be reassuring. Share, learn, and grow together.

By actively managing postpartum emotions through these strategies, you empower yourself to navigate the emotional landscape of motherhood with resilience and grace. Remember, your emotional well-being is an ongoing journey, and embracing these practices contributes to a positive and fulfilling postpartum experience.

3.2. SEEKING SUPPORT:

Building a strong support system, including partner, family, and friends.

Building a strong support system is a cornerstone of navigating the complexities of the postpartum period. This section explores the importance of seeking support from your partner, family, and friends, offering insights into fostering meaningful connections that contribute to your emotional well-being.

- **Partner Support:**

Your partner plays a pivotal role in your postpartum journey. Open communication is key—share your thoughts, emotions, and any challenges you may be facing. Discuss expectations and collaborate on caregiving responsibilities. A united front ensures that both you and your partner feel supported and understood.

- **Family Involvement:**

Engage your extended family in the postpartum experience. Grandparents, siblings, and other relatives can provide valuable assistance, whether it's helping with household tasks, caring for the baby, or offering emotional support. Communicate your needs and involve family members in a way that enhances the overall well-being of your growing family.

- **Friends as Allies:**

Lean on your circle of friends for emotional support. True friends are there to lend a listening ear, share experiences, and provide encouragement. Stay connected with those who uplift you and understand the unique challenges and joys of new motherhood.

- **Community of Moms:**

Joining a community of fellow moms creates a space for shared experiences and understanding.

Attend local mom groups or connect with online communities where you can exchange advice, share stories, and offer and receive support. The camaraderie of other moms can be immensely comforting.

- **Open Communication:**

Effective support hinges on open communication. Clearly express your needs, concerns, and feelings to those in your support network. This fosters understanding and ensures that your support system is aligned with your evolving requirements.

- **Delegating Responsibilities:**

Delegation is a powerful tool in managing postpartum demands. Entrust specific responsibilities to members of your support system. Whether it's meal preparation, household chores, or running errands, sharing the load allows you to focus on your recovery and bonding with your baby.

- **Setting Boundaries:**

While seeking support is crucial, setting boundaries is equally important. Clearly communicate your limits and make sure your support system understands when to offer assistance and when to give you space. Establishing these boundaries protects your well-being and promotes a healthy dynamic with your support network.

- **Expressing Gratitude:**

Expressing gratitude reinforces the bonds within your support system. Acknowledge the contributions of your partner, family, and friends. A simple thank you or a heartfelt expression of appreciation strengthens connections and fosters a positive and supportive environment.

- **Professional Support:**

In some instances, seeking professional support may be necessary. Mental health professionals, lactation consultants, and postpartum doulas are valuable resources. Don't hesitate to include these experts in your support network when needed.

- **Flexibility and Adaptability:**

Recognize that your support system may need to adapt to changing circumstances. Flexibility is key in navigating the evolving needs of your family. Be open to adjustments and communicate openly as your postpartum journey unfolds.

By actively cultivating a robust support system, you create a foundation of strength and resilience for your postpartum well-being. The bonds forged with your partner, family, and friends contribute to a nurturing environment where you can thrive as a new mother. Remember, seeking support is a sign of strength, and building these connections enhances the richness of your postpartum experience.

3.3. MENTAL HEALTH:

Strategies for maintaining good mental health, including mindfulness and stress management techniques.

Maintaining good mental health is essential during the postpartum period, and this section explores effective strategies, including mindfulness and stress management techniques, to support your mental well-being.

- **Mindfulness Practices:**

Incorporate mindfulness into your daily routine. Whether through meditation, deep breathing exercises, or mindful moments throughout the day, these practices help center your mind, reduce stress, and enhance overall well-being.

- **Establishing a Routine:**

Create a structured routine that includes time for self-care, rest, and activities that bring you joy. A well-defined routine provides a sense of predictability and control, contributing to a more stable mental state.

- **Setting Realistic Expectations:**

Manage expectations and avoid the pressure of perfection. Understand that your daily achievements, no matter how small, contribute to your overall well-being. Embrace the imperfections of motherhood, recognizing that it's okay not to have everything figured out.

- **Effective Stress Management:**

Develop a toolkit of stress management techniques. This may include exercise, creative outlets, or engaging in activities that bring you relaxation. Experiment with different approaches to discover what resonates best with you.

- **Quality Sleep:**

Prioritize quality sleep as it profoundly impacts mental health. Create a sleep-friendly environment, establish a bedtime routine, and enlist the support of your partner or family to ensure you get adequate rest.

- **Open Communication:**

Maintain open communication with your partner, friends, and family about your mental health. Sharing your thoughts and feelings fosters understanding and provides an outlet for emotional expression.

- **Professional Support:**

If needed, seek professional support from a mental health provider specializing in maternal well-being. Therapy can be a valuable resource for navigating the emotional challenges of postpartum life.

- **Me Time:**

Carve out dedicated time for yourself regularly. Whether it's a short break for a cup of tea, a solo walk, or indulging in a hobby, "me time" is essential for recharging and maintaining mental equilibrium.

- **Connect with Other Moms:**

Build connections with other moms who can empathize with your experiences. Sharing stories, advice, and support in a community of mothers fosters a sense of belonging and reduces feelings of isolation.

- **Reflective Journaling**:

Consider keeping a reflective journal to document your thoughts and emotions. Journaling provides a constructive outlet for self-expression and allows you to gain insights into your mental well-being.

- **Balanced Nutrition:**

A well-balanced diet contributes not only to physical health but also to mental well-being. Ensure your nutrition includes a variety of nutrient-rich foods that support brain function and overall vitality.

- **Celebrate Small Wins:**

Acknowledge and celebrate small victories. Each day presents new challenges and triumphs, and recognizing your achievements—no matter how modest—builds a positive mindset.

Remember, maintaining good mental health is an ongoing process, and these strategies can be tailored to fit your unique needs. Prioritize self-care, seek support when needed, and embrace a holistic approach to nurturing your mental well-being during the postpartum period.

CHAPTER 4:
SELF-CARE RITUALS

Welcome to the exploration of self-care, a chapter dedicated to the art of prioritizing "me time" and cultivating rituals that enhance your well-being. From simple beauty routines to strategies for restful sleep, this chapter guides you in creating a sanctuary of self-care amidst the beautiful chaos of motherhood.

4.1.   PRIORITIZING "ME TIME":

Creating space for self-care amidst the demands of motherhood.

In the whirlwind of motherhood, prioritizing "me time" is not just a luxury; it's a vital investment in your well-being. This section explores the art of creating space for self-care, providing strategies to nurture your mind, body, and soul amidst the demands of caring for a newborn.

- **Understanding the Importance of "Me Time":**

Acknowledge that taking time for yourself is not selfish; it's a fundamental component of maintaining balance and resilience. By prioritizing "me time," you recharge your energy, enhance your emotional well-being, and cultivate a positive mindset.

- **Carving Out Moments in Your Schedule:**

Identify pockets of time within your daily routine where you can dedicate moments to self-care. Whether it's during nap times, with the support of a partner, or through brief breaks, intentionally carving out these moments ensures that self-care becomes an integral part of your day.

- **Defining Your Self-Care Rituals:**

Discover what self-care means to you. It could involve activities such as reading, taking a soothing bath, practicing mindfulness, or enjoying a cup of tea. Define rituals that resonate with your preferences and bring you a sense of joy and relaxation.

- **Communicating Your Needs:**
Communicate openly with your partner, family, or support system about your need for "me time." Expressing your needs ensures that those around you understand the importance of these moments and can provide the support necessary for you to take them.

- **Creating a Self-Care Sanctuary:**
Designate a space in your home as a self-care sanctuary. It could be a cozy corner, a reading nook, or a spot where you can engage in activities that bring you solace. This space serves as a visual reminder to prioritize your well-being.

- **Incorporating Quick Self-Care Rituals:**
Recognize that self-care doesn't always require extended periods. Embrace quick rituals, such as deep breathing exercises, stretching, or a short

meditation session, that can be seamlessly integrated into your daily routine.

- **Outsourcing Tasks When Possible:**

Delegate tasks that can be handled by others to free up time for yourself. Whether it's household chores, grocery shopping, or other responsibilities, outsourcing allows you to focus on activities that replenish your energy.

- **Balancing "Me Time" with Social Connections:**

Combine self-care with social connections by engaging in activities that bring you joy with friends or family. This dual-purpose approach ensures that you satisfy both your need for solitude and your desire for social interaction.

- **Embracing Flexibility:**

Recognize that the concept of "me time" evolves as your circumstances change. Be flexible in adapting your self-care rituals to align with the demands of different phases of motherhood, allowing for a dynamic and sustainable approach.

- **Celebrating Small Victories:**

Acknowledge and celebrate each moment of "me time" as a small victory. Whether it's a few quiet minutes with a book or a brief walk outdoors, these moments accumulate to create a positive impact on your overall well-being.

By prioritizing "me time," you embark on a journey of self-nourishment and rejuvenation. This intentional practice not only benefits you but also enhances your ability to navigate the challenges of motherhood with resilience and joy. Remember, taking care of yourself is a profound act of love, both for yourself and for those you care for.

4.2. BEAUTY AND PAMPERING:

Simple self-care routines to boost confidence and well-being.

Embracing beauty and pampering rituals is a delightful avenue to boost confidence and enhance overall well-being. This section introduces simple yet effective self-care routines tailored to nourish your body, rejuvenate your spirit, and cultivate a sense of inner radiance amidst the demands of motherhood.

- **Morning and Evening Skincare Rituals:**
Establish a morning and evening skincare routine that caters to your skin's needs. Embrace cleansing, moisturizing, and, if time allows, indulge in a gentle facial massage. These rituals not only nurture your skin but also create moments of relaxation.

- **Quick and Effective Makeup Tips:**
Discover quick and effective makeup tips that enhance your natural beauty. Even with minimal time, a touch of mascara, a swipe of tinted

moisturizer, or a pop of blush can uplift your mood and boost confidence.

- **Hair Care for Self-Love:**

Treat your hair with care and indulge in simple hair care rituals. Whether it's a nourishing hair mask, a gentle scalp massage, or styling your hair in a way that makes you feel good, these practices contribute to both the health of your hair and your overall well-being.

- **At-Home Spa Experience:**

Transform your bathroom into a sanctuary with an at-home spa experience. Draw a warm bath, add soothing essential oils, and pamper yourself with a body scrub or a hydrating face mask. This immersive experience provides relaxation and rejuvenation.

- **Expressive Nail Care:**

Express yourself through nail care. Even a quick manicure or a coat of your favorite nail polish can be a simple yet effective way to indulge in self-care and add a touch of beauty to your daily routine.

- **Comfortable and Stylish Wardrobe Choices:**

Select wardrobe choices that make you feel comfortable and stylish. Investing time in choosing outfits that align with your personal style enhances your confidence and elevates your mood throughout the day.

- **Daily Affirmations and Mirror Moments:**

Incorporate daily affirmations while engaging in mirror moments. Stand in front of the mirror, appreciate your reflection, and affirm positive thoughts about yourself. This practice promotes self-love and boosts your overall sense of well-being.

- **Aromatherapy for Relaxation:**

Integrate aromatherapy into your daily routine. Whether through scented candles, essential oil diffusers, or fragrant lotions, select calming scents that promote relaxation and elevate your mood.

- **Gentle Exercise for Body and Mind:** Engage in gentle exercise routines that simultaneously care for your body and mind. Practices like yoga or Pilates not only contribute to physical well-being but also offer moments of mindfulness and tranquility.

- **Self-Reflection During Pampering:** Use pampering moments as an opportunity for self-reflection. Whether it's during a skincare routine or a quiet moment with a cup of tea, reflect on your journey, express gratitude for yourself, and celebrate the strength that resides within you.

By incorporating these simple beauty and pampering rituals into your routine, you infuse daily life with moments of self-love and care. These practices not only enhance your physical well-being but also contribute to the radiance that comes from embracing and celebrating the unique beauty that is inherently yours.

4.3. SLEEP HYGIENE:

Strategies for getting restful sleep and managing sleep deprivation.

Navigating the challenges of sleep is a crucial aspect of postpartum well-being. This section provides practical strategies for enhancing sleep hygiene, ensuring restful sleep, and managing sleep deprivation during this transformative period.

- **Creating a Sleep-Friendly Environment:**

Designate your bedroom as a peaceful and comfortable sleep haven. Adjust room temperature, use blackout curtains, and invest in a supportive mattress and pillows. These elements contribute to a conducive sleep environment.

- **Establishing a Consistent Sleep Schedule:**

Set a consistent sleep schedule by going to bed and waking up at the same time each day, even on weekends. This helps regulate your body's internal clock and improves the quality of your sleep over time.

- **Prioritizing a Bedtime Routine:**

Develop a calming bedtime routine to signal to your body that it's time to wind down. This may include activities such as reading a book, practicing gentle stretches, or enjoying a soothing cup of caffeine-free tea.

- **Limiting Screen Time Before Bed:**

Reduce exposure to screens at least an hour before bedtime. The blue light emitted by electronic devices can interfere with the production of the sleep hormone melatonin, making it harder to fall asleep.

- **Managing Nighttime Feedings:**
If you're breastfeeding, consider a bedside bassinet or co-sleeping arrangement to minimize disruptions during nighttime feedings. Streamlining this process can help you and your baby return to sleep more easily.

- **Delegating Nighttime Responsibilities:**
Share nighttime responsibilities with your partner or a support person. Having someone take turns with nighttime feedings or diaper changes can ensure that the burden is not solely on one person, promoting more restful sleep for both.

- **Napping Strategically:**
Incorporate strategic napping into your routine. Short naps (20-30 minutes) can provide a quick energy boost without disrupting nighttime sleep. Aim to nap earlier in the day to avoid interference with your nighttime sleep.

- **Mindful Sleep Positions:**

Experiment with different sleep positions to find the most comfortable and supportive option. Utilize pillows to provide additional support for breastfeeding or to alleviate discomfort, especially if recovering from a cesarean section.

- **Seeking Assistance When Needed:**

If sleep deprivation becomes overwhelming, don't hesitate to seek assistance. Enlist the help of family or friends to provide support during particularly challenging nights, allowing you to get much-needed rest.

- **Practicing Relaxation Techniques:**

Incorporate relaxation techniques into your bedtime routine. Deep breathing exercises, progressive muscle relaxation, or guided meditation can help calm your mind and promote a restful transition into sleep.

- **Hydration and Nutrition Awareness:**

Be mindful of hydration and nutrition. While staying hydrated is important, try to limit excessive fluid intake close to bedtime to minimize nighttime bathroom trips. Consider a light, balanced snack if hunger is a concern.

- **Professional Guidance if Needed:**

If sleep challenges persist, consider seeking guidance from healthcare professionals. A consultation with your healthcare provider or a sleep specialist can provide personalized advice tailored to your specific situation.

By implementing these sleep hygiene strategies, you can create an environment conducive to restful sleep, manage sleep deprivation more effectively, and promote overall well-being during the postpartum period. Remember, prioritizing your sleep is a valuable investment in your physical and emotional health as you navigate the joys and challenges of new motherhood.

CHAPTER 5:
BONDING WITH BABY

Welcome to a chapter dedicated to the profound and heartwarming journey of bonding with your newborn. Explore tips for nurturing a strong connection and discover the joy of enhancing this bond through the soothing touch of baby massage and engaging activities that create moments of shared joy.

5.1. NURTURING CONNECTION:

Tips for fostering a strong bond with your newborn.

Building a strong bond with your newborn is a heartwarming journey filled with moments of connection and love. Here are tips to help you foster a deep and meaningful bond with your precious little one:

- **Skin-to-Skin Contact:**

Embrace the power of skin-to-skin contact. Spend dedicated time cuddling with your baby, allowing the warmth and closeness to create a deep emotional connection. This practice is not only comforting but also supports your baby's physical and emotional well-being.

- **Eye Contact and Smiles:**

Engage in frequent eye contact and share smiles with your baby. These simple yet powerful gestures create a foundation for communication and emotional connection. Your gaze communicates love and establishes a sense of security.

- **Responsive Parenting:**

Practice responsive parenting by promptly attending to your baby's cues. Whether it's feeding, changing, or comforting, meeting your baby's needs fosters a sense of security and trust. Responding with warmth and attentiveness builds a strong foundation for a secure attachment.

- **Narrate Your Day:**

Share your daily experiences with your baby. Narrate your activities, sing lullabies, or read stories aloud. Your voice becomes a comforting presence, and the rhythm of your words creates a familiar and soothing environment. This verbal interaction contributes to language development and strengthens your bond.

- **Baby-Wearing Bond:**

Explore the practice of baby-wearing. Using a baby carrier or wrap allows you to keep your baby close while going about daily activities, promoting a sense of security and attachment. The physical closeness enhances your connection and allows your baby to experience the world from the comfort of your embrace.

- **Create a Routine:**

Establish a daily routine that includes special bonding moments. Whether it's a morning cuddle, a bedtime ritual, or a special playtime, routines provide predictability and comfort, strengthening the bond between you and your baby.

- **Be Present During Feedings:**
Whether breastfeeding or bottle-feeding, use feeding times as opportunities for bonding. Maintain eye contact, talk softly, and cherish these moments of closeness. The nurturing act of feeding creates a strong emotional connection between you and your baby.

- **Gentle Touch and Caresses:**
Incorporate gentle touches and caresses into your interactions. Stroke your baby's soft skin, hold their tiny hands, and provide comforting touches. Physical contact is a powerful way to convey love and establish a secure attachment.

- **Engage in Face-to-Face Interaction:**
Regularly engage in face-to-face interactions with your baby. Make funny faces, mimic their expressions, and observe their reactions. This playful engagement fosters connection and enhances your understanding of each other.

- **Practice Patience and Presence:**
Cultivate patience and be fully present during your interactions. Babies respond to the calm and reassuring presence of their caregivers. By being attentive and patient, you create an environment where your baby feels secure and loved.

Building a strong bond with your newborn is a gradual and beautiful process. Each of these tips contributes to the rich tapestry of connection that forms between you and your baby. Cherish the small moments, be attuned to your baby's needs, and savor the joy of nurturing a bond that will continue to grow and evolve over time.

5.2.   BABY MASSAGE AND GENTLE ACTIVITIES:

Enhancing the bond through soothing touch and engaging activities.

Discover the joy of deepening your bond with your baby through the art of baby massage and gentle activities. These tender interactions not only provide soothing touch but also create meaningful moments of shared joy and connection:

- **Introduction to Baby Massage:**

Embark on the journey of baby massage. Use gentle, loving strokes to massage your baby, starting with their legs and arms and gradually incorporating their chest, back, and belly. This tactile experience fosters relaxation and strengthens your emotional connection.

- **Sensory Play and Exploration:**

Engage your baby in sensory play. Introduce soft fabrics, varied textures, and gentle toys for exploration. This sensory-rich environment stimulates your baby's senses and offers delightful moments of interaction.

- **Mirror Play:**

Introduce mirror play to your baby. Position a baby-safe mirror in front of them and observe their reactions as they discover their reflection. This simple activity encourages self-recognition and provides an opportunity for shared play.

- **Tummy Time Fun:**

Make tummy time enjoyable. Use colorful mats, soft toys, and your engaging presence to create a positive tummy time experience. This activity not only strengthens your baby's muscles but also provides an opportunity for shared play.

- **Baby Talk and Singing Sessions:**

Engage in frequent baby talk and singing sessions. Your baby delights in the cadence of your voice, and these interactions contribute to language development while fostering a joyful bond. Sing lullabies, nursery rhymes, or even make up your own songs.

- **Gentle Movement and Rocking:**
Incorporate gentle movements and rocking into your daily routine. Whether swaying to music or gently rocking your baby in your arms, these rhythmic motions provide comfort and create moments of connection. Rocking can also be incorporated during feeding or before bedtime.

- **Bath Time Bonding:**
Transform bath time into a bonding experience. Use soothing baby-friendly products, maintain eye contact, and engage in gentle play during baths. This routine becomes a cherished moment of connection and relaxation.

- **Baby Yoga and Stretching:**
Explore gentle baby yoga and stretching exercises. Gently move your baby's arms and legs in a way that mimics natural movements. These activities promote flexibility, muscle development, and create opportunities for interaction.

- **Soft Touch and Caresses:**

Continue to incorporate soft touches and caresses into your daily interactions. Run your fingers gently over your baby's skin, cradle them in your arms, and provide loving touches during moments of care. This physical connection nurtures a sense of security.

- **Engage in Peek-a-Boo:**

Play the classic game of peek-a-boo with your baby. Cover your face with your hands and then reveal it with a smile. This simple game delights babies and enhances their visual tracking skills, while also creating moments of shared laughter.

- **Soft Rattles and Musical Toys:**

Introduce soft rattles and musical toys during playtime. The gentle sounds and textures capture your baby's attention, creating a multisensory experience that adds joy to your shared moments.

- **Nature Walks and Outdoor Strolls:**
Take leisurely nature walks or gentle outdoor strolls with your baby. The sights, sounds, and fresh air provide a stimulating and calming environment, fostering a connection with the world around them and creating opportunities for shared exploration.

By incorporating these gentle activities into your daily routine, you not only enhance your baby's physical and cognitive development but also create a bond built on love, trust, and shared joy. These moments of connection contribute to the foundation of a strong and enduring relationship with your precious little one.

As you embark on this journey of bonding with your baby, savor each moment of connection and embrace the unique ways in which your relationship blossoms. Whether through nurturing touch, shared smiles, or engaging activities, the bond you cultivate lays the foundation for a lifetime of love and connection between you and your precious little one.

CHAPTER 6:
BALANCING RESPONSIBILITIES

Juggling the responsibilities of motherhood, work, and personal time requires effective time management. Explore strategies to maintain balance and make the most of your time:

6.1. TIME MANAGEMENT: JUGGLING MOTHERHOOD, WORK, AND PERSONAL TIME EFFECTIVELY.

Effectively managing your time as a mother juggling various responsibilities requires strategic planning and prioritization. Explore practical strategies to maintain balance and make the most of your precious time:

- **Prioritize Your Tasks:**

Identify and prioritize tasks based on their urgency and importance. This helps you focus on what truly matters, ensuring that essential responsibilities are addressed first.

- **Establish a Daily Routine:**

Create a daily routine that includes dedicated time blocks for different aspects of your life—motherhood, work, and personal activities. Having a structured routine provides predictability and helps manage your time more efficiently.

- **Set Realistic Expectations:**

Set realistic expectations for what you can accomplish in a given day. Acknowledge that as a mother with multiple responsibilities, some days may be busier than others. Be kind to yourself and celebrate small victories.

- **Utilize Time-Blocking Techniques:**

Implement time-blocking techniques to allocate specific time periods for different tasks. Designate focused work hours, dedicated childcare time, and intervals for personal activities. This approach minimizes multitasking and enhances productivity.

- **Leverage Technology:**
Explore productivity tools and apps to help streamline tasks and keep you organized. Calendar apps, to-do lists, and task management tools can be invaluable in managing your schedule and staying on top of deadlines.

- **Combine Activities When Possible:**
Look for opportunities to combine activities efficiently. For example, engage in activities with your child that align with your personal interests, or integrate work-related tasks that allow you to spend quality time with your family.

- **Delegate Responsibilities:**
Delegate tasks when possible. Whether it's household chores, work-related responsibilities, or childcare duties, share the workload with your partner, family members, or trusted individuals within your support network.

- **Embrace Flexibility:**

Cultivate flexibility in your schedule. Recognize that unexpected events may arise, and being adaptable allows you to navigate changes without feeling overwhelmed. Embracing flexibility is key to managing the dynamic nature of motherhood and work.

- **Prioritize Self-Care:**

Allocate dedicated time for self-care. Whether it's a short break, exercise, or pursuing a hobby, prioritizing self-care is essential for maintaining your well-being and sustaining the energy needed for both motherhood and work.

- **Set Boundaries:**

Establish clear boundaries between work and personal time. Communicate your work hours to colleagues and family, and set limits on when you are available for work-related tasks. This helps create a balance between your professional and personal life.

- **Learn to Say No:**

Recognize your limitations and be comfortable saying no when necessary. Overcommitting can lead to burnout, so prioritize tasks and commitments that align with your goals and values.

- **Reflect and Adjust:**

Regularly reflect on your time management strategies and adjust them as needed. Life circumstances and priorities may change, so being adaptable and willing to reassess your approach ensures continued effectiveness.

Balancing motherhood, work, and personal time is an ongoing process that requires thoughtful planning and flexibility. By implementing these time management strategies, you can create a harmonious and fulfilling lifestyle that meets both your professional and personal needs.

6.2. DELEGATING AND ACCEPTING HELP:

Building a support network and sharing responsibilities.
Delegating and Accepting Help: Building a Support Network and Sharing Responsibilities

Creating a support network and effectively sharing responsibilities is crucial for maintaining balance and well-being as a mother. Here are practical strategies for delegating tasks and accepting help:

- **Identify Your Support System:**

Identify individuals within your support system who can offer assistance. This may include your partner, family members, friends, or even neighbors. Recognize that building a reliable support network is a collaborative effort.

- **Communicate Your Needs Clearly:**

Openly communicate your needs and challenges to those in your support system. Clearly express how others can assist you, whether it's with childcare, household tasks, or emotional support. Effective communication is key to building a collaborative network.

- **Delegate Specific Tasks:**

Delegate specific tasks to individuals within your support network. Assign responsibilities based on their strengths and availability. Whether it's sharing household chores or seeking help with childcare, distributing tasks lightens the load for everyone involved.

- **Share Parenting Responsibilities:**

If you have a partner, establish a shared parenting approach. Collaborate on childcare responsibilities, including feeding, diaper changes, bedtime routines, and playtime. Shared parenting fosters a sense of teamwork and strengthens your bond as parents.

- **Accept Help Gracefully:**

Learn to accept help gracefully. Understand that accepting assistance is not a sign of weakness but a practical choice to manage responsibilities effectively. Allow others to contribute to your well-being and the well-being of your family.

- **Rotate Responsibilities:**

Rotate responsibilities among family members or support individuals. Distributing tasks ensures that no one person bears the entire burden, and everyone has an opportunity to contribute to the well-being of the family.

- **Set Clear Expectations:**

When delegating tasks, set clear expectations regarding timelines and specific requirements. Clear communication helps prevent misunderstandings and ensures that tasks are completed in a manner that aligns with your needs.

- **Express Gratitude:**

Express gratitude to those who support you. Acknowledge and appreciate the contributions of your support network. Gratitude fosters positive relationships and encourages ongoing collaboration.

9. Be Open to Different Approaches:
Recognize that others may have different approaches to tasks. Be open to varying methods and appreciate the effort put forth by those assisting you. Flexibility in accepting help strengthens your support network.

- **Seek Professional Support When Needed:**

Consider seeking professional support when needed. This could include hiring a babysitter, utilizing daycare services, or engaging professionals for specific tasks. Professional support can provide additional resources to help balance responsibilities.

- **Create a Supportive Community:**

Build a community of like-minded individuals who understand the challenges of motherhood and can offer empathy and advice. Join parenting groups, online communities, or local meet-ups to share experiences and resources.

- **Establish Regular Check-Ins:**

Establish regular check-ins with your support network. Regular communication ensures that everyone is on the same page regarding responsibilities and allows for adjustments as needed. A collaborative approach promotes a sense of shared responsibility.

Building a strong support network and sharing responsibilities is a dynamic process that evolves as your circumstances change. By implementing these strategies, you cultivate a foundation for a supportive community that enhances your well-being and enables you to navigate the complexities of motherhood more effectively.

CHAPTER 7:
RELATIONSHIP DYNAMICS

7.1. NURTURING YOUR PARTNERSHIP:

Strategies for maintaining a healthy relationship with your partner during this transformative time.

Maintaining a healthy relationship with your partner during the transformative period of motherhood is crucial. Explore strategies to nurture your partnership amid the joys and challenges:

- **Prioritize Quality Time:**

Despite busy schedules, prioritize quality time with your partner. Whether it's a simple date night, a quiet evening at home, or a shared activity, dedicating time to each other strengthens your connection.

- **Foster Open Communication:**

Create a space for open and honest communication. Discuss your feelings, concerns, and joys. Effective communication is the cornerstone of a healthy relationship, especially during significant life changes.

- **Share Parenting Responsibilities:**
Collaborate on parenting responsibilities. A shared approach to childcare fosters teamwork and ensures that both partners contribute to the well-being of the family. Acknowledge each other's efforts and support one another in your parenting roles.

- **Express Gratitude:**
Regularly express gratitude for each other. Acknowledge the small gestures, the support given, and the effort put into managing the challenges of parenthood. Gratitude cultivates a positive and appreciative atmosphere.

- **Keep Intimacy Alive:**
Prioritize intimacy in your relationship. While the demands of parenthood can be intense, finding moments for physical and emotional connection is essential. Communicate your needs and maintain a sense of closeness.

- **Be Flexible and Patient:**

Recognize the need for flexibility and patience. Understand that both partners may be adjusting to new roles and responsibilities. Approach challenges with a collaborative mindset and be patient as you navigate this transformative time together.

- **Seek Support Together:**

If needed, seek support together. Whether it's through couples counseling, parenting classes, or connecting with other couples going through similar experiences, seeking support as a team strengthens your bond.

- **Maintain Individual Identities:**

While building a shared life, maintain individual identities. Nurture your personal interests and hobbies. This not only enriches your own life but also brings diversity and vitality to your relationship.

- **Create Rituals and Traditions:**

Establish rituals and traditions that are unique to your partnership. Whether it's a weekly movie night, a special meal, or an annual getaway, these shared experiences create lasting memories and deepen your connection.

- **Be Mindful of Each Other's Well-Being:**

Prioritize each other's well-being. Be attuned to your partner's needs and emotions. Supporting each other's emotional health is integral to maintaining a strong and resilient partnership.

7.2. COMMUNICATING NEEDS:

Open communication and understanding each other's roles.

Open communication and understanding each other's roles are foundational for a thriving partnership. Explore effective ways to communicate needs and navigate the evolving dynamics:

- **Schedule Regular Check-Ins:**

Establish regular check-ins to discuss your individual needs and concerns. These conversations create a dedicated space for open dialogue and ensure that both partners feel heard and understood.

- **Be Clear About Expectations:**

Communicate your expectations openly. Discuss each other's roles, responsibilities, and expectations in the context of parenthood. Clarity prevents misunderstandings and fosters a shared understanding of your evolving roles.

- **Express Emotions Honestly:**

Encourage honest expression of emotions. Share your feelings, fears, and joys with your partner. Creating a safe space for emotional vulnerability strengthens your connection and fosters mutual understanding.

- **Use "I" Statements:**

When expressing needs or concerns, use "I" statements to convey your feelings without placing blame. For example, say "I feel overwhelmed when..." rather than "You always..."

- **Practice Active Listening:**

Practice active listening during conversations. Give your partner your full attention, and validate their feelings and perspectives. This ensures that both partners feel respected and valued in the relationship.

- **Be Empathetic:**

Cultivate empathy towards your partner's experiences. Understand that the challenges of parenthood may impact each partner differently. Empathy creates a supportive environment where both individuals feel understood.

- **Adapt Communication Styles:**
Recognize and adapt to each other's communication styles. Some individuals may prefer direct communication, while others may need time to process before discussing certain topics. Being attuned to these differences enhances effective communication.

- **Collaboratively Problem-Solve:**
Approach challenges as a team and collaboratively problem-solve. Work together to find solutions that address both partners' needs. A collaborative mindset strengthens the sense of unity in your partnership.

- **Be Flexible in Roles:**
Be flexible in adapting to evolving roles. Parenthood may bring about changes in responsibilities, and flexibility allows both

partners to share the load in a way that suits the family's needs.

- **Celebrate Achievements:**

Celebrate each other's achievements, no matter how small. Acknowledge the efforts made in managing the demands of parenthood and maintaining a healthy partnership. Celebrations reinforce positive dynamics in the relationship.

By nurturing your partnership and fostering open communication, you create a resilient foundation for navigating the complexities of parenthood together. These strategies contribute to a strong and enduring relationship that supports both partners on their journey through this transformative time.

CHAPTER 8:
PLANNING FOR THE FUTURE

8.1. CAREER AND PERSONAL GOALS:

Balancing motherhood with personal and professional aspirations.

Balancing the multifaceted roles of motherhood with personal and professional aspirations is an intricate journey. Navigate this path with these strategic approaches:

- **Define Clear Priorities:**

Establish clear priorities for both motherhood and personal/professional goals. This clarity forms the foundation for making informed decisions and managing your time effectively.

- **Set Realistic and Achievable Goals:**

Define realistic and achievable goals for your career and personal life. This ensures a balanced approach to pursuing your aspirations while considering the demands of motherhood.

- **Open Communication with Your Employer:**

Maintain open communication with your employer about your career aspirations and potential adjustments needed. Discuss flexible work arrangements to harmonize your professional responsibilities with your role as a mother.

- **Explore Remote Work Opportunities:**

Explore remote work options if applicable to your job. Remote work can provide the flexibility needed to fulfill your professional commitments while actively participating in your child's life.

- **Efficient Time Management:**

Refine your time management skills to balance work and motherhood demands. Prioritize tasks, set boundaries, and optimize your schedule to maximize productivity without compromising personal and family time.

- **Continuous Professional Development:**
Continue investing in your professional development. Engage in online courses, workshops, and networking opportunities to stay connected with your career goals and evolving industry trends.

- **Collaborative Parenting with Your Partner:**
Collaborate with your partner to share parenting responsibilities. A supportive partnership allows both individuals to pursue personal and professional goals, fostering a sense of balance and fulfillment.

- **Embrace Flexibility:**
Embrace flexibility in adjusting your goals as circumstances evolve. Parenthood often brings unexpected challenges, and a flexible mindset allows you to adapt your plans while staying true to your overarching objectives.

8.2. LONG-TERM SELF-CARE:

Sustainable practices for ongoing well-being beyond the early postpartum period.

Sustaining well-being beyond the initial postpartum period involves intentional, long-term self-care practices. Explore strategies for maintaining health and happiness over the years:

- **Prioritize Mental Health:**

Make mental health a priority by incorporating mindfulness and stress management techniques into your daily routine. Cultivating emotional well-being is crucial for long-term resilience.

- **Establish Consistent Self-Care Rituals:**

Create consistent self-care rituals aligned with your needs and sources of joy. Daily walks, reading, or dedicated quiet time contribute to sustained well-being over the years.

- **Cultivate and Maintain Social Connections:**
Cultivate and maintain meaningful social connections. Nurturing relationships with friends and family provides emotional support and a sense of community, contributing to overall well-being.

- **Schedule Regular Health Check-Ups:**
Prioritize regular health check-ups to monitor and address any health concerns proactively. Proactive health management is a key element of long-term well-being.

- **Set Clear Boundaries:**
Establish clear boundaries to protect your time and energy. Learning to say no when necessary and creating space for rest are essential components of sustained well-being.

- **Engage in Hobbies and Interests:**
Engage in hobbies and interests outside of motherhood. Pursuing activities that bring

personal fulfillment contributes to a sense of well-rounded identity and long-term happiness.

- **Embrace Continuous Learning:**
Cultivate a mindset of continuous learning. Whether through reading, attending classes, or acquiring new skills, staying intellectually engaged contributes to ongoing personal growth.

- **Financial Planning for Long-Term Stability:**
Include financial planning in your long-term self-care strategy. Building a secure financial foundation enhances peace of mind and contributes to long-term stability.

- **Regular Reflective Practices:**
Incorporate regular reflection on your goals and aspirations. This practice allows for ongoing assessment and adjustment of priorities, ensuring alignment with your evolving self.

- **Embrace Aging with Grace:**

Approach the aging process with grace and acceptance. Embracing the natural changes that come with aging fosters a positive and resilient mindset for the years ahead.

By incorporating these strategies into your life, you lay the groundwork for a future that balances the demands of motherhood with your personal and professional aspirations, contributing to a fulfilling and well-rounded journey.

CHAPTER 9:
SLEEP STRATEGIES FOR NEW MOMS

Welcome to the sleep-focused chapter of "New Mum Self-Care Book." In this chapter, we delve into essential tips and strategies to optimize sleep patterns for both you and your baby. From coping with inevitable sleep deprivation to establishing healthy sleep routines, we explore ways to enhance the quality of your rest and promote overall well-being.

9.1.   TIPS FOR OPTIMIZING SLEEP PATTERNS FOR BOTH YOU AND YOUR BABY.

<u>For Your Baby:</u>

- **Establish a Consistent Sleep Routine:**

Create a calming bedtime routine for your baby. This might include activities like a warm bath, gentle massage, or reading a bedtime story. Consistency helps signal that it's time for sleep.

- **Create a Comfortable Sleep Environment:**

Ensure the sleep environment is conducive to rest. Maintain a comfortable room temperature, use soft bedding, and consider white noise to drown out disturbances.

- **Encourage Daytime Naps:**

Help your baby establish healthy sleep patterns by encouraging regular naps during the day. A well-rested baby is more likely to sleep better at night.

- **Differentiate Day and Night:**

During daytime feedings and interactions, keep the environment bright and engage with your baby. In the evening, dim the lights and keep noise levels low to signal that it's nighttime.

- **Respond to Your Baby's Cues:**

Learn your baby's sleep cues and respond promptly. This helps prevent overtiredness, making it easier for your baby to settle into sleep.

For You:

- **Nap When Your Baby Naps:**

Prioritize rest during the day by napping when your baby sleeps. This can help offset nighttime wake-ups and ease the effects of sleep deprivation.

- **Share Nighttime Responsibilities:**

If possible, work with your partner to share nighttime responsibilities. Taking turns with feedings and soothing can ensure both parents get adequate rest.

- **Create a Relaxing Bedtime Routine:**

Establish a calming bedtime routine for yourself. This might involve activities like reading a book, taking a warm bath, or practicing relaxation exercises to signal your body that it's time to wind down.

- **Limit Screen Time Before Bed:**

Reduce exposure to screens at least an hour before your planned bedtime. The blue light emitted by screens can interfere with the production of the sleep hormone melatonin.

- **Prioritize Sleep Hygiene:**

Ensure your sleep environment is conducive to rest. Keep the bedroom dark, quiet, and at a comfortable temperature. Invest in a comfortable mattress and pillows for quality sleep.

- **Accept Help:**

Don't hesitate to accept help from friends and family. Having support with household tasks or someone to watch the baby can provide you with valuable time for rest.

Remember, each baby is unique, and it may take some time to establish consistent sleep patterns. Be patient with yourself and your baby as you navigate this adjustment, and don't hesitate to seek advice from pediatricians or sleep specialists if needed.

9.2. COPING WITH SLEEP DEPRIVATION AND ESTABLISHING HEALTHY SLEEP ROUTINES.

Coping with sleep deprivation and establishing healthy sleep routines is crucial for both you and your baby. Here are some tips:

<u>Coping with Sleep Deprivation:</u>
- **Prioritize Sleep:**

When possible, prioritize sleep over non-essential tasks. A well-rested parent is better equipped to handle the challenges of caring for a baby.

- **Take Short Naps:**

Embrace short naps to help combat sleep deprivation. Even a 20-30 minute nap can provide a quick energy boost.

- **Accept Help:**

Don't be afraid to ask for and accept help. Whether it's a family member, friend, or partner, having support can make a significant difference.

- **Create a Support System:**

Build a network of supportive friends or fellow new parents. Sharing experiences and advice can provide emotional support during challenging times.

- **Practice Mindfulness:**

Incorporate mindfulness techniques into your daily routine. Short meditation sessions or deep-breathing exercises can help manage stress and improve overall well-being.

Establishing Healthy Sleep Routines:

- **Consistent Bedtime Routine:**

Establish a consistent bedtime routine for both you and your baby. A routine signals that it's time for sleep, helping your baby learn when to expect bedtime.

- **Set a Regular Sleep Schedule:**

Aim to set a regular sleep schedule for both you and your baby. Consistency helps regulate your body's internal clock, making it easier to fall asleep and wake up at the desired times.

- **Limit Stimulating Activities Before Bed:**

Reduce exposure to bright lights and stimulating activities at least an hour before bedtime. This can include avoiding screens and engaging in calming activities instead.

- **Create a Relaxing Environment:**

Make your sleep environment conducive to rest. Dim the lights, keep the room cool, and use white noise if needed. Consider blackout curtains to minimize external light.

- **Be Flexible and Patient:**

Recognize that sleep routines may need adjustments over time. Be flexible and patient as your baby grows and their sleep patterns evolve. It's a gradual process.

Remember, every baby is different, and what works for one may not work for another.

Consistency and patience are key when establishing healthy sleep routines. If challenges persist, consult with your pediatrician or a sleep specialist for personalized advice based on your baby's unique needs.

9.3. CREATING A CALMING BEDTIME ROUTINE FOR IMPROVED SLEEP QUALITY.

In this section, we explore the importance of a calming bedtime routine for both you and your baby. Establishing a peaceful pre-sleep ritual contributes to improved sleep quality, setting the stage for restful nights and enhanced well-being.

<u>For Your Baby:</u>
- **Warm Bath:**

Begin the routine with a warm bath for your baby. The soothing water can help relax muscles and create a calming transition to bedtime.

- **Gentle Massage:**

Follow the bath with a gentle massage using baby-friendly lotion or oil. This tactile experience fosters a sense of comfort and relaxation.

- **Soft Music or Lullabies:**

Play soft, calming music or lullabies as part of the bedtime routine. Music has a calming effect and can become a signal that it's time for sleep.

- **Dim the Lights:**

Lower the lights in the room as bedtime approaches. Dim lighting helps signal the body to produce melatonin, the hormone responsible for sleep.

- **Read a Bedtime Story:**

Incorporate a short bedtime story into the routine. The rhythmic nature of your voice can be soothing, creating a positive association with sleep.

For You:

- **Create a Relaxing Atmosphere:**

Dim the lights in your bedroom to signal that it's time to wind down. Consider using soft, neutral colors for bedding and decor to create a serene atmosphere.

- **Limit Screen Time:**

Reduce exposure to screens at least an hour before your planned bedtime. Engage in activities that promote relaxation, such as reading a book or practicing gentle stretches.

- **Practice Relaxation Techniques:**

Incorporate relaxation techniques into your routine, such as deep-breathing exercises or gentle yoga stretches. These activities help calm the mind and prepare your body for sleep.

- **Disconnect from Electronic Devices:**

Avoid using electronic devices like phones or tablets right before bed. The blue light emitted by screens can interfere with the production of melatonin.

- **Set a Regular Bedtime:**

Establish a consistent bedtime for yourself. A regular sleep schedule helps regulate your body's internal clock, promoting better sleep quality.

A calming bedtime routine is a powerful tool for improving sleep quality for both you and your baby. By creating a peaceful environment and engaging in soothing activities, you set the stage for restful nights and a more rejuvenated start to each day. Sweet dreams await as you embrace the tranquility of bedtime rituals.

CHAPTER 10:
ESTABLISHING SELF-CARE ROUTINES

In this chapter, we explore the art of establishing self-care routines tailored to the unique demands of motherhood. From developing a personalized self-care plan to finding moments of relaxation, mindfulness, and joy, we delve into strategies for creating a harmonious balance between the needs of your baby and your own well-being.

10.1. DEVELOPING A PERSONALIZED SELF-CARE PLAN THAT FITS INTO YOUR DAILY LIFE.

Developing a personalized self-care plan that seamlessly fits into your daily life is crucial for maintaining overall well-being during the demands of motherhood.

Here's a step-by-step guide to help you create a plan tailored to your unique needs:

- **Self-Assessment:**

- Reflect on your physical, emotional, and mental well-being.

- Identify areas that need attention or improvement.

- Consider activities that bring you joy and relaxation.

- **Set Realistic Goals:**

- Establish achievable self-care goals that align with your current lifestyle.

- Break down large goals into smaller, manageable steps.

- Prioritize goals based on your immediate needs and long-term aspirations.

- **Create a Schedule:**

- Allocate specific times for self-care activities in your daily or weekly schedule.

- Treat these appointments with the same importance as other commitments.

- Be flexible and willing to adapt your plan as needed.

- **Prioritize Sleep:**

- Recognize the importance of sufficient sleep for overall well-being.

- Establish a bedtime routine that promotes relaxation.

- Consider short naps or rest periods during the day to replenish energy.

- **Identify Quick Self-Care Practices:**

- Pinpoint short and simple self-care practices you can incorporate into your daily routine.

- Examples include deep breathing, stretching, or enjoying a brief moment of quiet reflection.

- **Incorporate Enjoyable Activities:**

- Integrate activities you genuinely enjoy into your self-care plan.

- Whether it's reading, listening to music, or engaging in a hobby, make time for what brings you joy.

- **Leverage Micro-Moments:**

- Find joy in small, everyday moments with your baby.

- Savor a smile, a giggle, or a quiet cuddle as moments of connection and happiness.

- **Practice Mindful Breaks:**
- Incorporate mindful breaks throughout the day.
- Pause for a few moments to focus on your breath or observe the present without distraction.

- **Regular Check-Ins:**
- Periodically assess your self-care plan and adjust as needed.
- Be aware of changes in your needs and circumstances, and adapt your plan accordingly.

- **Seek Support:**
- Share your self-care goals with your partner, family, or friends.
- Seek their support in creating an environment that fosters your well-being.

Remember, your self-care plan is a dynamic and evolving tool. It should be adaptable to the changing demands of motherhood. Regularly revisit and adjust your plan, ensuring that it remains a positive and sustainable part of your daily life.

10.2. FINDING MOMENTS FOR RELAXATION, MINDFULNESS, AND JOY AMIDST THE DEMANDS OF MOTHERHOOD.

- **Mindful Morning Moments:**

- Begin your day with a few minutes of mindfulness. Take slow, intentional breaths and set positive intentions for the day ahead.

- **Naptime Mindfulness:**

- During your baby's naptime, indulge in a short mindfulness practice. This could be guided meditation, deep breathing exercises, or simply savoring a moment of quiet.

- **Nature Connection:**

- Spend time outdoors with your baby. Whether it's a stroll in the park or sitting in the backyard, connect with nature for a refreshing break.

- **Joyful Playtime:**

- Engage in joyful playtime with your baby. Participate in activities that bring laughter and smiles, fostering a positive connection.

- **Quick Relaxation Breaks:**

- Identify short breaks throughout the day for quick relaxation. Close your eyes, stretch, or practice a mini-meditation to release tension.

- **Mindful Feeding:**

- Use feeding times as an opportunity for mindfulness. Focus on the sensory experience, the connection with your baby, and the nourishment being provided.

- **Gratitude Journaling:**

- Maintain a gratitude journal. Take a few minutes each day to jot down things you're grateful for, shifting your focus toward positive aspects of your life.

- **Self-Care Snippets:**

- Integrate self-care snippets into your routine. Even a few minutes of self-care, such as applying lotion, can be rejuvenating amidst daily tasks.

- **Mindful Movement:**

- Incorporate mindful movement into your routine. This can be a gentle yoga stretch, a short dance break, or a mindful walk with your baby.

- **Technology-Free Time:**

- Designate technology-free moments. Put away your phone and be fully present with your baby, fostering a deeper connection and reducing external distractions.

- **Mindful Evening Reflection:**

- End your day with a mindful reflection. Acknowledge your achievements, express gratitude, and let go of any stressors from the day.

- **Bedtime Rituals:**

- Create calming bedtime rituals for both you and your baby. This could include a soothing lullaby, dimmed lights, and a moment of quiet connection before sleep.

Remember, finding moments for relaxation, mindfulness, and joy doesn't require large chunks of time. Embrace the simplicity of these practices, and weave them organically into your daily routine. These moments of self-care contribute to your well-being amidst the beautiful chaos of motherhood.

10.3. BALANCING THE NEEDS OF YOUR BABY WITH YOUR OWN WELL-BEING.

- **Establish Realistic Expectations:**

- Recognize that balancing a baby's needs with your own requires flexibility. Set realistic expectations for what you can accomplish each day.

- **Prioritize Self-Care:**

- Understand that taking care of yourself is essential for being the best caregiver for your baby. Prioritize self-care as an integral part of your routine.

- **Delegate Responsibilities:**

- Enlist the support of your partner, family, or friends. Delegate responsibilities to share the load, ensuring you have time for self-care and rest.

- **Communication with Your Partner:**
   - Maintain open communication with your partner about your needs and feelings. Discuss how you can support each other in balancing parenting responsibilities and personal well-being.

- **Baby-Friendly Self-Care:**
   - Explore self-care activities that involve your baby. This could include baby-wearing walks, gentle exercises together, or simply enjoying quiet moments of connection.

- **Create a Support System:**
   - Build a support system of friends or fellow parents. Share experiences, advice, and provide mutual support to navigate the challenges of motherhood.

- **Set Boundaries:**
   - Establish boundaries to protect your personal time. Communicate your self-care needs to those around you, ensuring that you have the space to prioritize your well-being.

- **Time Management:**

- Efficiently manage your time by prioritizing tasks. Identify essential activities and allocate time for self-care, maintaining a balance between caregiving and personal needs.

- **Quality over Quantity:**

- Focus on the quality of your interactions with your baby rather than the quantity. Meaningful moments of connection contribute to a strong bond.

- **Listen to Your Body:**

- Pay attention to your body's signals. If you need rest, take a break. If you're feeling overwhelmed, ask for help. Listening to your body is crucial for overall well-being.

- **Celebrate Small Wins:**

- Acknowledge and celebrate small achievements. Whether it's completing a task or finding time for self-care, celebrate these victories as they contribute to a positive mindset.

- **Flexible Routine:**
    - Embrace a flexible routine that accommodates both your needs and your baby's. Adjustments may be necessary as your baby grows, ensuring the routine remains supportive for both of you.

Balancing the needs of your baby with your own well-being is an ongoing process that requires self-awareness and adaptability. By nurturing your own health and happiness, you enhance your ability to provide the best care for your baby.

CONCLUSION

As we conclude this guide, **"NEW MUM SELF CARE BOOK,"** we reflect on the transformative journey you've embarked upon. Motherhood is a multifaceted adventure, and this book aims to be your companion, offering guidance on self-care and thoughtful planning for the future.

Throughout the chapters, we delved into the intricacies of embracing the transition into motherhood, acknowledging the changes—both physical and emotional—that accompany this profound experience. We explored the landscape of emotions, provided practical advice for postpartum recovery, and offered insights into nourishing nutrition and gentle fitness tailored for new moms.

In the realm of self-care, we emphasized the importance of prioritizing "me time," indulging in beauty and pampering routines, and understanding the significance of sleep hygiene. We recognized the essential bond between you and your baby, providing tips on nurturing connection through activities like baby massage and gentle play.

The book extended beyond the immediate postpartum period, venturing into the complexities of balancing responsibilities—mastering time management and building a strong support system. We addressed the significance of maintaining good mental health, seeking support, and implementing strategies for self-care rituals amidst the demands of motherhood.

The exploration continued into the dynamics of relationships, focusing on nurturing partnerships and fostering open communication. As you plan for the future, we offer insights into harmonizing career and personal goals, sustaining well-being through long-term self-care practices, and setting the stage for a fulfilling and balanced life.

In the heart of this guide is the recognition that motherhood is a dynamic journey, one that evolves with each passing day. It's a journey of self-discovery, resilience, and continuous growth. As you navigate the challenges and celebrate the joys, remember that self-care is not a luxury but a necessity—a foundation upon which you can build a flourishing future for both yourself and your family.

May this guide serve as a source of inspiration and practical wisdom, offering support as you navigate the beautiful tapestry of motherhood. As you nurture your well-being, cultivate meaningful relationships, and plan for the future, may you find fulfillment and joy in every step of this extraordinary journey.

Wishing you strength, love, and abundant joy on your path of nurturing motherhood.

www.ingramcontent.com/pod-product-compliance
Lightning Source LLC
Chambersburg PA
CBHW070947260726
48661CB00003B/1166